Chronic Stress and Illness

"Some *people make remarkable recoveries from serious,*
and even life-threatening, diseases or dangerous surgery,
but other seemingly similar people succumb -they become
more debilitated or die. In many cases, it seems that the
only major difference between success and failure abstruse
quality of the patient known as the will to live" (Friedman,
2001). Chronic illness can be described as the irreversible
deterioration of the body that leaves a patient unable to
return to a health state of being. The subconscious is
known to control all of our bodily processes and behaviors;
the beliefs and thoughts we hold will affect all aspects of
our well-being. Fear and negative emotion in the
subconscious can cause energy blocks that that will either
contribute to or intensify chronic pain and illness. People
are often not aware of the factors that are contributing to

intensifying their pain or illness because these factors are hidden in the subconscious mind, where the flow of healthy energy is blocked from allowing the body to heal (Beck, nd).

The autonomic nervous system provides almost instantaneous communication between the brain and other organs. The sympathetic nervous system will mobilize the body by increasing heart rate and preparing the body to either fight or flee as the parasympathetic nervous system will restore the body to its natural state (Friedman, 2001). Over-activation of the sympathetic nervous system can pose a serious risk to the body as the heart rate increases and the blood pressure rises too rapidly. As the body begins to slow down, over-activation of the parasympathetic nervous system will cause exhaustion, resulting in the body giving up or shutting down. The hypothalamus of the brain is responsible for hormone regulation and metabolism. As it influences bodily functions, the pituitary glands will secrete hormones that influence other endocrine organs. When the adrenal glands are activated, the adrenal cortex will secrete steroid hormones that will have negative effects on the body. As the sympathetic nervous system secretes the hormones epinephrine and norepinephrine, these substances enter the blood stream and travel throughout the body causing increased arousal during severe threats.

The neurotransmitter serotonin is responsible for regulating mood, sleep, pain, and eating. Low levels of serotonin can be contributed to clinical depression, mood, and eating disorders. As the fight or flight response is triggered by psychological and physical threats, stressful life events may produce continuous bodily arousal. In turn, this can cause lasting changes in the psychological process. General adaptation syndrome consists of three stages and consists of alarm reaction, resistance, and exhaustion (Friedman, 2001). As negative responses develop as a result of unpleasant stimuli, various organs are affected. It is possible that various diseases may result due to prolonged adaptive processing. Since stress will lower bodily resistance, chronic stresses can lead to excessively high or low levels of cortisol, which will suppress the immune system.

Chronic stress will cause the physiological systems to work overtime and become strained. Allostatatic load refers to the stress responses being repeatedly turned off and on; resulting in physical bodily damage. Although genes may play a significant role in determining the general biological tendency to good health and a healthy immune system, factors such as environmental influences, thoughts, feelings, and behaviors will also drastically affect human health and development. Life events have also been known to drastically impact respiratory, gastrointestinal, and cardiovascular systems. More diseases are now being viewed as having a psychosomatic component, meaning that various diseases are in part caused by physiological factors, such as stress. Since stress involves the nervous and endocrine system, these systems must prepare the body for environmental changes while they maintain internal balance. These changes are directly dependent on the nervous system. As stress may alter these functions, the impact will result in the deterioration of physical health.

The Connection to Mental and Physical Health

It is the perception of health that influences behaviors associated with either poor or strong health. It is through interactions with others that the self-concept develops, which influence the behaviors that determine overall health status. Emotions and thought patterns can also drastically impact one's health, playing a direct role in the recovery rate amongst patients. Descartes' Dualism describes the mind and body as being separate, but very closely related entities. Although some tried to merge the two together, others argued that the body existed only within the mind. Although it's difficult to conceive the mind and body as one entity, it does seem strong seem to individuate that the mind, which directly influences behaviors, will play a concrete role in determining the life style that will influence one's physical health. As lifestyle and behaviors such as diet and exercise, will influence physical health and immune system functioning, unhealthy behaviors can be contributed to both social and personal factors. Maintaining a healthy body is somewhat under the control of the individual, with abuses of the body being closely related to problems of self-image. It is the social influences that will either encourage or discourage the self-image, habits, and lifestyle of the individual.

Correlation verses causation refers to the factors that cause an illness and its relationship between certain behaviors (Friedman, 2001). In understanding the relationship between the two, attempts can be made to prevent and/or treat the illness. However, the conclusions do not always give clear indications between the behaviors that cause illness, and the illnesses which may influence specific behaviors, such as heightened stress. For instance, stress can cause a number of illnesses, such as heart disease and high blood pressure, but many people also experience heightened stress due to the specific illness. As these negative feelings may also slow down recovery rates, poor recovery and treatment may increase the levels of stress. Heightened levels of stress may also influence negative behaviors, such as smoking and/or substance abuse. As life stressors may trigger these behaviors, it is these behaviors that trigger negative physical effects on the body, which in turn cause life-threatening illnesses and disease.

The immune system is in place to protect the body from invading bacteria and abnormal cells, such as cancer or viral invasions. A recent study published in 1977, looked at the effects of bereavement on the immune system, this study brought attention to the link between stress and illness or disease (Friedman, 2009). Although immune functioning cannot be contributed to disease, an immune system that is completely dysfunctional will increase the likelihood of various diseases or illnesses occurring. As behavior will play a role in the functioning of the immune system, positive behaviors, such as maintaining a healthy diet and regular exercise, can be used to help maintain healthy immune functioning. In order for cells in the body to function and reproduce, they need glucose, nutrients, and oxygen, as well as being free from wastes and other toxins. So in order to promote a healthy internal environment, factors such as proper nutrition, healthy heart and lung functioning, and a healthy circulatory system must be in place.

Free radicals are molecules that have an imbalance in their electrical charge causing damage to healthy cells. Maintaining healthy cells can be contributed to proper levels of glucose in the blood. Glycogenesis involves breaking down glycogen into glucose through enzymes that are regulated by nerves and hormones (Friedman, 2009). As stress hormones help establish proper glucose levels in the blood, stress can upset this process, which in turn can affect one's physical health. This indicates there is a direct connection between stress and a healthy immune system. In order to maintain a healthy immune system, healthy cells must also be maintained through proper glucose levels. Positive behaviors, such as maintaining a healthy diet, eliminating stress, and regular exercise can significantly increase glucose levels and help support healthy immune functioning. Toxic substances, such as alcohol and other substances, can hinder healthy cell functioning and hinder the immune and circulatory systems.

Chronic stress may cause the physiological systems to over work and become strained. Allostatatic load refers to the stress responses being repeatedly turned off and on and the physical damage it may cause. Although genes may play a significant role in determining the health and immune system of an individual's, thoughts, feelings, and behaviors may also drastically affect human health and development. Life events have also been known to have an effect on the respiratory, gastrointestinal, and cardiovascular systems. More diseases are now being viewed as having a psychosomatic component, meaning that various diseases are in part caused by physiological factors such as stress (Friedman, 2001). Since stress involves the nervous and endocrine system, these systems must prepare the body for environmental changes and maintain internal balance. These changes depend on the nervous system. As stress may alter these functions, it seems this may also have a significant impact on physical health.

Stable mental health seems to play a direct role in the behaviors which will result in positive physical health as mental and physical health seems to offset the other. In order to maintain a consistent and well-balanced internal environment, we must maintain healthy cell function. Keeping our cells healthy means we need to keep our cells at a healthy temperature while supplying our bodies with certain energy, such as food, water, and oxygen (Friedman, 2009). As emotional conflicts may play a role in various diseases or illnesses, our bodies must also be equipped to constantly adjust to meet the body's changing demands

(Friedman, 2009). Although our behaviors and lifestyles may alter our immune system and physical health, positive behaviors may also produce positive effects on the immune system and overall bodily functioning. Emotions and thought patterns may also directly play a role in the choices and behaviors that contribute to either positive or negative effects on the body. So the link between stress, behavior and lifestyle, mental health, and physical health and illness, although separate entities, are all interrelated in determining an individual's health status.

Addiction, Illness, and Recovery

In chronic illnesses such as addiction, the mind also plays a crucial role in the addiction process. The brain of an addict differs from the brains of those who are not addicted. Scientific evidence shows us that addicted brains are damaged. Addiction is often coupled with other mental disorders that must be treated simultaneously (Hoffman, 2007). When a person relapses due to an addiction, part of this illness is directly the manifestation of a mental illness, since many addicts are not only physically addicted, but psychologically addicted as well. Relapses in addictive illnesses do not significantly differ from those rates in other illnesses (Buddy, 2010). The potential for relapse is a part of any chronic disease, and addiction is no different. Just as people with chronic diseases must adjust their lifestyle and assume responsible for managing their own care, the same is true in those with addictions to drugs and alcohol. Recovery from alcohol and other drugs is a process of change in which an individual achieves abstinence and improved health, wellness and quality of life (Kipins & Killar, nd). Like many chronic illnesses, an addicted individual cannot return to his or her previous psychological state since recovery is continuous. Treatment for addiction should not solely focus on abstinence, but should also incorporate improvements in other areas of life, such as family relationships and employment. The goal with treating addiction is to put the illness into remission; treatment should be an ongoing process.

Since some individuals consume drugs and alcohol for the purpose of self-treatment for emotional pain, high stress levels are also linked to substance abuse problems. The multiple consequences of substance abuse suggest that stress levels are very high among active users. Patients with substance abuse addictions are most likely to transition to recovery when they have shown high levels of self-help group participation, lowered levels of stress, and have a support network in place. Addiction, like any other chronic illness, requires a certain level of social support in order for the addict to reestablish their pre-addictive identities. Support from family, along with other support groups, can offer encouragement and a greater sense of identity. Unlike many other chronic illnesses, such as cancer or heart disease, there is a negative stigma attached to addiction, which may hinder the desire to seek treatment and plague the recovery process. Criticism from family and friends will more than likely leave an individual suffering from addiction feeling frustrated and misunderstood. This level of stress and frustration actually may encourage relapses from well-meaning family members, so it is important to be surrounded by those who emulate understanding and encouragement. By providing emotional support, the addict can begin to surround him or herself with a positive social network that will be beneficial to acquiring a new sense of identity and crucial for the recovery process.

Any genuine recovery process consists of a number of critical steps. The first step of addiction recovery involves overcoming denial. Individuals who seek treatment must accept the necessity in changing patterns of addictive behavior (Addiction Recovery Process, 2010). Support groups, which offer social and emotional support, are also a necessary means for the addict to regain a positive outlook. Through support groups, the addict can form a new circle of friends and should refrain from previous social groups that may also struggle with substance abuse. The next step involves checking into a rehabilitation center in order to ensure a safe and managed withdrawal. The addict may need to continue treatment in a residential, outpatient or inpatient rehabilitation center depending on the severity of the addiction (Addiction Recovery Process, 2010).

Recovery is a lifelong process, so continuous support is crucial in the journey to recovery. To ensure progress, addicts should learn to recognize the warning signs of a relapse. Healthy and positive substitutes should be chosen in place of the problematic substance. Support groups should be maintained, and contact with enablers should be reduced (Addiction Recovery process, 2010). The importance of social support on influencing behavior are crucial in indirectly influencing behavior, reducing stress;

and through providing assistance, emotional support, and a sense of belonging which will improve overall life satisfaction. Evidence has linked social support to increased health, happiness, and longevity. Substance users with lower levels of social support are also more likely to relapse. Recovery-oriented support may also help supply a greater level of self-efficiency toward ongoing abstinence because it allows recovering addicts to acquire effective coping strategies through their peers (Laudet, Morgen, & White, 2006).

Spirituality and Healing

Spirituality and religion can play a major role in the recovery process for many individuals suffering from any form of chronic illness. Awareness of a higher spiritual power seems to be the foundation for many recovering from addiction, illness, or disease. Spirituality, faith, and religion can offer a sense of peace, hope, and belonging; all components to improved health and recovery. Scientific evidence strongly supports the notion that spirituality and religion can enhance an individual's health and quality of life. In a review involving more than 200 studies, positive relationships were documented with physical and functional status, reduced psychopathology, greater emotional well-being, and improved methods of coping (Laudet, Morgen, & White, 2006). Stress is also often cited as one of the major causes of relapse in physical illness and addiction. Individuals who have a strong sense of religious faith tend to have greater levels of life satisfaction, lower levels of stress, and tend to have better coping skills and greater levels of recovery when facing a chronic illness.

As spirituality and religion seems to provide higher levels of resiliency in stressful situations, it also seems to link lower levels of substance abuse in those with strong religious faith. A recent study indicates that religiosity reduced the impact of life stress on initial level of substance use and on rate of growth in substance use over time (Laudet, Morgen, & White, 2006). Protective mechanisms conferred by religious involvement may include avoidance of drugs, social support advocating abstinence or moderation, alternative activities that are incompatible with drug use, and promotion of pro-social values that promote a drug free lifestyle. Numerous research supports the notion that religion and spirituality may enhance the likelihood of attaining and maintaining recovery from addiction or physical illness and disease. Individuals recovering from sickness or addiction often report that religion and spirituality was a critical factor in their recovery process. Long-term studies have also indicated that there is a link between increased religious involvement and remission among addicts and those suffering from terminal illness. Furthermore, evidence suggests that high levels of religious faith in recovering addicts and those with physical illness can be linked to greater overall health outcomes, with higher levels of resilience to stress, lower levels of anxiety, and positive coping skills.

Positive Mental Health, Illness and Recovery

Stable mental health will play a direct role in the behaviors that affect overall physical well-being. As positive physical and mental health seems to offset the other, tending to one and not the other would be fruitless and counterproductive. In order to maintain a consistent and well-balanced internal environment, we must maintain healthy cell function. Keeping our cells healthy means we need to keep our cells at a healthy temperature while supplying our bodies with certain energy, such as food, water, and oxygen. As emotional conflicts may play a role in various diseases and illnesses, our bodies must also be equipped to constantly adjust to meet the body's changing demands. Although behaviors and lifestyles may alter the immune system and impact physical health, positive behaviors can also produce positive effects on the immune system while boosting overall bodily functioning. Emotions and thought patterns directly play a role in the choices and behaviors that will contribute to either positive or negative effects on the body. So the link between stress, behavior and lifestyle, mental and physical health, and illness; although separate entities, are all interrelated in determining an individual's overall health status.

There is no doubt that pain can be caused by physical problems, but physical pain is also greatly impacted by parts of the brain involving perception, emotion, motivation, and action (Friedman, 2001). Chronic illness and addiction recovery will involve the physical, mental, and emotional aspects of the individual. In order to recovery to be the most successful, the recovering individual must nurture the mind and body as a whole. Social support, emotional support, and religious faith seem to set the foundation for recovering health, well-being, and life satisfaction. Higher levels or life satisfaction and lower levels of stress seem to create an overall sense of identity and wellness. It is through these encouraging factors that an individual is able to acquire the coping skills necessary for the journey to recovery. All of these factors all play a role in the subconscious, which controls behaviors, thoughts, and emotions. As the body the mind and body work together in the healing process, the recovering individual will have fewer relapses and a greater chance of overall recovery and increased wellness.

Psychosocial Crisis and Life Stage Development

Erik Erikson's theory of integrity verses despair examines the various aspects that play a role in the levels of resiliency and wellness as throughout life. As an individual moves throughout the course of their life from infancy to late adulthood, eight distinct stages of development will occur. Successful completion of each stage will produce a positive sense of self and high feelings of self-worth. However, interruptions during one of these stages may result in unresolved crisis; negatively affecting an individual's sense of self-worth, life satisfaction, and overall health status. Erikson's theory that supports resolution of one psychosocial crisis stage being dependent on successful resolution of subsequent stages, allows for further assessment and a deeper analogy of the psychosocial crisis of integrity verses despair that occurs during later adulthood.

Erikson's *Theory of Psychosocial Development* emphasizes eight distinct stages of development, with two possible outcomes occurring. According to this theory, successful completion of each stage will result in a positive sense of self and successful social interactions with others. Failure to complete a stage can reduce the ability to complete further stages, resulting in an unhealthy sense of self (Psychology 101, 2002). As each psychosocial crisis stage is dependent on successful resolution of previous stages, subsequent stages will be influenced according to the resolutions, or lack of resolution that occur (Krauss-Whitbourne, et.al., 1992). Feelings of purposelessness, hopelessness, or chronic stress will trigger the psychosocial crisis of integrity verses despair, which can directly impact physical health. According to this theory, when an individual's productivity slows down, personal evaluations of usefulness will occur. Integrity will develop if a sense of accomplishment is gained. However, feelings of guilt about the past, or viewing the past as unproductive, may result in dissatisfaction with life or feelings of despair and hopelessness. Assessing the entire family unit and learning more about personal family history can allow additional issues to be examined. Problems of external origin that derive from conflicts or internal problems, such as depression, denial, and frustration, may hinder the ability to recognize the need for help (Ries, M.D. 2012). Medical issues can trigger feelings of hopelessness, which may further aggravate feelings of depression and despair.

The psychosocial crisis, integrity verse despair, involves life review, introspection, and self-evaluation. Contemporary factors, such as health, family relationships, and role loss or role transition are integrated with the assessment of past aspirations and accomplishments (Newman & Newman, 2012). Integrity can be described as the ability to accept the facts of one's life and face death without fear while reconciling life events. The attainment of integrity is a result of the balance of the psychosocial crisis that came early in life, accompanied by ego strengths and core pathologies that have accumulated throughout the course of one's life. When a sense of integrity is established, the ability to integrate past history with present circumstances produces contentment with the outcome. An individual, who lacks strong feelings of integrity, may have various regrets that have occurred throughout life. One theory, created by Neil Krause, describes a four-measure of meaning of life, which include: (1) having a system of values, (2) having a sense of purpose, (3) having goals to strive for, and (4) and reflecting on the past to reconcile past accomplishments with goals (Newman & Newman, 2012). Although there may be specific goal-sets and accomplishments that have occurred through the course of a life, lacking a sense of purpose may occur with the diagnosis of an illness. These factors can create feelings of anxiety and depression. Without social and emotional support, levels of grief surrounding an illness will not be dealt with in a healthy manner, and will therefore further suppress recovery and healing.

When a person receives high levels of emotional support from friends and family members, higher levels of life meaning are achieved and preserved. Anticipated support can also play a role in the changes that take place in a person's sense of meaning and wellness. When and individual is confident they can count on others for emotional support, their sense of meaning is strengthened while feelings of trust and hope increase. Anxiety may also be further heightened due to conflict and pressure, making it far more likely to contribute to feelings of purposelessness and despair. In order to experience integrity, a person needs to be able to incorporate their self-image with a life-long record of conflicts, failure, disappointments, and accomplishments. They must then come to terms with the fact that some of their hopes for themselves may accomplished in their lifetime. During middle adulthood, the psychosocial crisis of generativity verses stagnation is described as the adult who is committed to improving the life conditions of future generations (Newman & Newman, 2012).

Although setting goals and achieving accomplishment during middle adulthood may contribute to levels of life-satisfaction, chronic illness can cause unnecessary feelings of stagnation. As physical functioning diminishes and levels of independence lessen, discouragement and feelings of low self-worth may become greater. These factors are likely to create feelings of regret about the past, a desire to be able to do things differently, or bitterness about how life has turned out (Newman & Newman, 2012). This combine with unresolved issues from the past surrounding the psychosocial crisis of generativity verses stagnation, can have a drastic negative affect concerning the feelings of having no purpose. In order to address these feelings, it may be necessary to go back to an earlier point in your life to assess stumbling blocks that may have previous led to feelings of stagnation. This can allow past issues to be resolved so they are not carried over and intertwined with current circumstance. This will allow

more effective methods of self-help to be implementing in

order to combat the issues surrounding current life

circumstances.

Improving Health and Wellness

A recent study that compared older adults in the United States and Holland indicates that within both cultures, attainment of social contact and family goals were the strongest predictors of overall life satisfaction (Newman & Newman, 2012). Life satisfaction and resiliency is supported through a sense of belonging, which may be lost while battling a chronic illness. Social relationships are a primary source of meaning. Those who experience loneliness or inadequate social networks are much less satisfied with life than those who perceive themselves as positively connected to a meaningful circle of loved ones and friends. Negative relationships and ongoing exposure to interpersonal conflict can disrupt feelings of life-satisfaction while suppressing the immune system and its ability to combat illness.

Issues such as memory loss and loss of physical abilities may also be aggravated by cultural and societal views regarding disability due to illness or addiction, and the general feelings of have a lack of purpose. Although this may pose as a challenge for people as they feel they have to constantly redefine themselves and prove their levels of self-worth, new patterns of thought that occurs can be used increase levels of resiliency. The limitations of formal operational reasoning can provide new methods of post-formal thought. This can be characterized through a greater reflection of self, personal values, and emotions, the ability to find solutions based on past experiences, and a willingness to examine conflicting thoughts while reflecting upon these experiences. Acquiring a flexible integration of cognition and emotion allows for adaptive, reality-oriented, and satisfying solutions to be implemented. Maintaining a mind-set that encompasses enthusiasm for seeking new questions, finding and solving new problems, and utilizing new frameworks for understanding experiences strengthens the ability to cope with life's stressors while increasing overall physical and mental wellness.

In order to reach heightened levels of resiliency and wellness, issues or circumstances that may have occurred as early as infancy or early childhood, must be evaluated to ensure the crisis does not continuously occur. Generational customs and cultural values regarding parenting styles, methods of communication and collaboration, discipline that occurred during early childhood, and feelings of support, may all need to be addressed in order to increase levels of wellness and the ability to cope with life changes. Achieving a sense of heightened integrity requires the ability to introspect about the gradual evolution of life events and appreciate their significance in the formation of the adult personality. This can be achieved through individual effort, which involves reminiscence of long-term memories and events and finding closure. These feelings and experiences can also be counteracted with new, positive values or ideals, such as high priorities in relation to wisdom and personal well-being. Through assessing each stage of the psychosocial developmental factors that played a role in shaping the sense of self, determinations regarding methods of treatment or lifestyle change can be better determined. The psychosocial crisis of integrity verses despair that occurs during middle adulthood may stem from a previous psychosocial crisis that was unresolved. As an individual learns to re-evaluate life accomplishment, a positive reflection of self will develop, contributing to greater feelings of integrity, self-worth, and resiliency.

Cognitive Restructuring for Improved Well-Being

In order to change the maladaptive thought patterns that directly impact wellness and physical functioning, goals to achieve new behaviors and thought patterns must be realistic and achievable. If the end result or desired behavior seems out of reach or overly difficult, an individual may be unaware of the appropriate steps needed in order to complete the desired task. Cognitive coping skills training may be needed in order to teach new cognitive behaviors that will be used to promote the desired behaviors. All-or-nothing thinking and overgeneralization may also be playing a role in the ineffectiveness of behavioral modification techniques. Don't fall victim to the mind-set that wants to make you believe that if the tasks carried out are not perfect, they are not acceptable. You may be under the belief that a single negative experience is evidence that something is all bad or is always going to be result in failure. Work toward new behavioral goals in small, realistic, and achievable steps and focus on your accomplishment, rather than your setbacks. In order to increase the likelihood that behavioral modification will produce positive results, cognitive restructuring may be used to identify behaviors you find distressing so that you can examine your past and current circumstances to get rid of these distressing thoughts while replacing them with more desirable thought patterns and self-talk.

Cognitive coping is a behavior modification procedure designed to teach new cognitive behaviors when an individual does not have the cognitive behaviors needed to cope effectively with problem situations or when behavioral deficits exist. Cognitive restructuring can be used in three basic steps: (1) identify the distressing thoughts and the situations in which they occur, (2) identify the emotional response, unpleasant mood, or problem behavior that follows the distressing thought, (3) don't dwell on distressing thoughts; instead replace those thoughts with more rational or desirable thoughts and behaviors (Miltenberger, 2008). This process of breaking down each step in the behavior chain into smaller steps will simplify the desired tasks, making them appear less threatening or overwhelming. This may also help eliminate any negative thoughts or emotional responses that are triggered. By learning to cope with each issue one step at a time as they occur, reinforcement will occur, making carrying out these activities more desirable.

Priming is often used by providing a stimulus in order to influence future thoughts and actions. Perceptual priming is based on the form of the stimulus, where part of the picture is completed based on what was earlier observed. Repetitive priming occurs when repetition leads to it influencing later thoughts (Changing Minds, 2011). Backwards chaining used with repetition can help give you the skills needed to complete the various processes involved with completing specific tasks aimed at creating new behaviors and thought patterns. This allows desired skill-sets to be acquired through a step-by-step approach. As personal reinforcement is used to encourage new behaviors and thoughts, bodily responses will began to change and become more productive and proactive in accordance to these newly found thought patters.

References

Addiction Recovery Process (2010). Retrieved January 14, 2011 from

http://www.treatment4addiction.com/recovery/#

Beck, E. (nd). New Directions, Mind Body Connection. Retrieved January 12,

    2011 from http://www.mind-body-connections.biz/

Buddy, T. (2010). Addiction Relapse Similar To Other Chronic Diseases.

    Retrieved January 13, 2011 from

    http://alcoholism.about.com/cs/relapse/a/blcaron030804.htm

Changing Minds (2011). Priming. Retrieved October 8, 2011 from

    http://changingminds.org/explanations/theories/priming.htm#So

Friedman, H.S. (2001). Health psychology (2nd ed.). Upper Saddle River, NJ:

    Prentice Hall.

Hoffman, J. (2007). Understanding Addiction. Retrieved January 13, 2011 from

    http://www.huffingtonpost.com/john-hoffman/understanding-

    addiction_b_44618.html

Kipins, S. MD, FACP, FASAM & Killar, R. CASAC (nd). Managing Addiction

    As A Chronic Disease. Retrieved January 13, 2011 from

    www.oasas.state.ny.us/AdMed/documents/mngngadctn.ppt

Laudet, A.B., PhD, Morgen, K. PhD, & White, W.L. MA (2006). The Role of

    Social Supports, Religiousness, Life Meaning and Affiliation with 12-

    Step Fellowships in Quality of Life

Miltenberger, R. (2008). Behavior Modification: Principles and Procedures,

    Fourth Edition. Wadsworth, Cengage Learning: Belmont, CA.

Satisfaction Among Individuals in Recovery from Alcohol and Drug Problems.

 Retrieved January 13, 2011 from

 http://www.ncbi.nlm.nih.gov/pmc/articles/PMC1526775/

Wilmot, W.W., Hocker, J. L. (2011). Interpersonal Conflict. Eighth Edition. New

 York, NY: McGraw-Hill Companies, Inc.

www.ingramcontent.com/pod-product-compliance
Lightning Source LLC
Chambersburg PA
CBHW020906310526
45786CB00018B/1896